Advanced Praise for *The Dynamic Dozen*

" *Straightforward, easy to read, and easy to implement! Tim Keim's book provides a practical approach to effectively help those of us diagnosed with osteoporosis. With clear explanations addressing much more than the physical effects on our bones, this book should be provided as a standard health care intervention.*"

— **Neil Pearson**, physical therapist, yoga therapist, founding chair of the Canadian Physiotherapy Pain Science Division

" *I'd show up to do this class with Tim. He knows his subject well and has chosen and explained very well a dozen asana to help any body, in particular those with osteopenia/osteoporosis. It's true that our three adult primary postures of standing, sitting, and lying reduce our strength, balance, and range of motion. Tim offers us* **relaxed exertion and comfortable engagement**. *I was ready to practice along as I was reading it. Here's a regular guy doing yoga — love the pictures — looks like my yoga practice. Tim shares how a simple practice for a few minutes per day makes our life more* **juicy** *and allows us to 'take delight in the massaging quality of the breath.' Sounds good to me — simply presented to keep our bones strong and flexible. Thanks for a caring, compassionate book, Tim.*"

— **Durga Leela**, founder of Yoga of Recovery and director of the Ayurveda Programs at the Yoga Farm in California

The Dynamic Dozen

12 accessible yoga poses for building bone density, strength, and balance

Tim Keim

LYSTRA BOOKS
& Literary Services

> The ideas, suggestions, and methods in this book are not intended to substitute for the advice of a trained medical professional. Consult your physician or medical professional about any condition that may require diagnosis or medical attention before adopting the suggestions in this book. The author and publisher disclaim any liability arising directly or indirectly from the use of this book.

The Dynamic Dozen: 12 Accessible Yoga Poses for Building Bone Density, Strength, and Balance
© Tim Keim 2014
All rights reserved

ISBN 978-0-9911502-5-0 print
ISBN 978-0-9911502-6-7 ebook
Library of Congress PCN 2014942481

Unless otherwise noted, all text is written by Tim Keim; its accuracy and originality are his responsibility.

Please respect the author's work. Except for short excerpts for reviews, no portion of this book may be reproduced in any medium without written permission of the author. He can be reached at **timkeim.wordpress.com**.

Cover and book design by Kelly Prelipp Lojk

Interior photography by Anky Chau, used by permission

Author's photograph by Jan Balster, used by permission

Published by Lystra Books and Literary Services, LLC

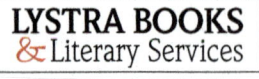

WWW.LYSTRABOOKS.COM

Published in the USA, 2014

*I dedicate the following pages to my students who inspired me
to write about their adventures in rebuilding their bones
and to those who will read these words and
be inspired by their victorious example.*

The Poses

The Standing Poses

Mountain 13
Warrior II 15
Warrior I 19
Tree 21
Dancer's Pose . . . 23
Warrior III 25
Triangle 27

The Sitting and Prone Poses

Cobra 31
Locust 37
Plank 39
Bridge 41
Boat 45
Yoga Sit-Ups 47
Savasana 49

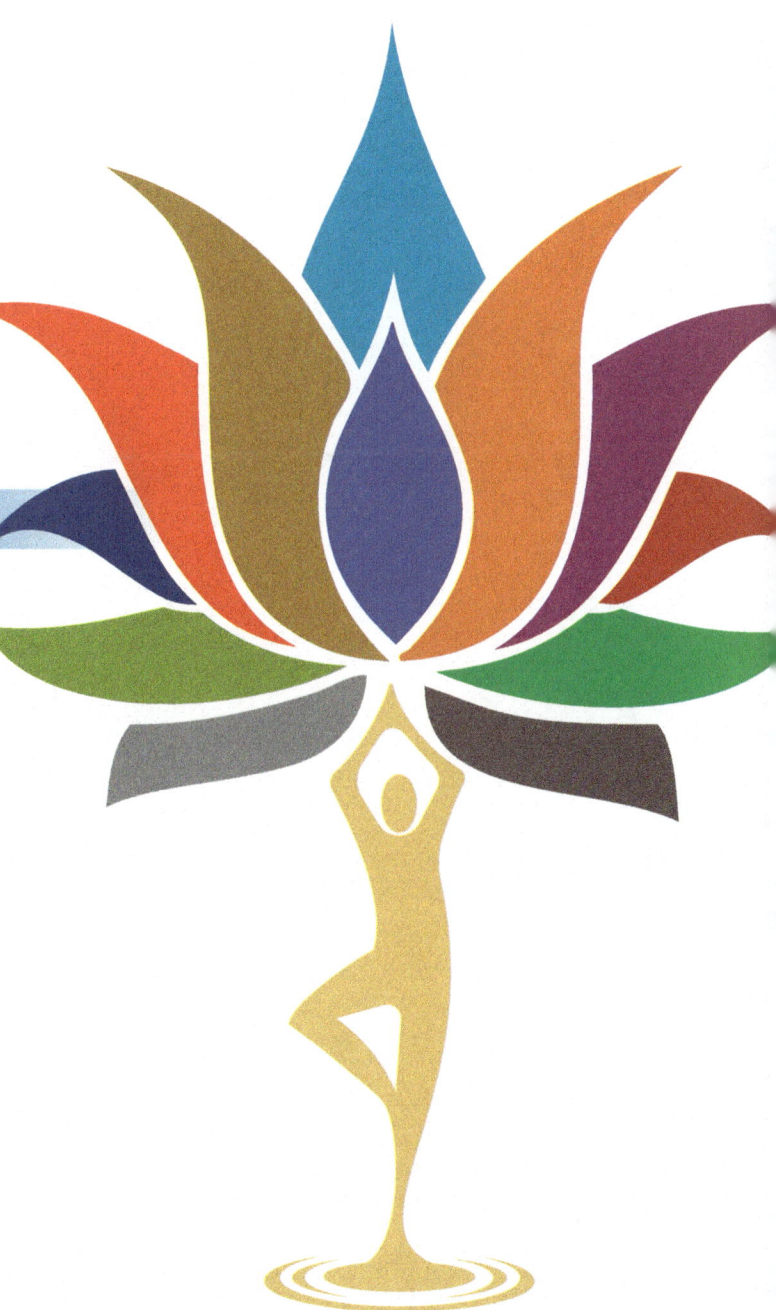

Introduction

One of the leading causes of debilitating injury and death among seniors is falling. Falling may result when seniors lose their sense of balance because of weakness caused by lack of exercise. When poor balance and osteoporosis coincide, this is a recipe for bone fractures.

The word *osteoporosis* comes from the Greek, *ostoun* meaning bones and *poros* meaning porous. You could picture it as having holes in your bones. Bone density refers to the concentration of bone tissue in any part of the skeleton. The most common type of bone thinning often occurs in women after menopause. Though this disease is found predominantly in women, it can also strike men.

Being diagnosed with osteoporosis or its precursor, osteopenia, is not an immutable sentence of progressive disease and disability. The truth of the matter is quite the opposite. The tools you need are at hand for you to rebuild your bone density and balance and to stake your claim on many more years of living in freedom and independence. The tools I'm talking about are inexpensive and can be used right in the comfort and privacy of your own home. They are the tools of Hatha Yoga.

Many people become less active as they age. Decreased activity weakens muscles and balance. Hatha Yoga practice, as you will see in the following pages, helps you to strengthen your muscles and your balance. Stronger muscles and balance will make falling much less likely. The weight-bearing exercises of Hatha Yoga will strengthen your muscles to help you reclaim your balance and rebuild your bone density.

Hatha Yoga is an ancient science that began thousands of years ago as an intuitive, common sense way for people to take care of their health and well-being. The practice flourished in India and is now known worldwide for its ability to address all questions of disease and healing.

New clinical studies are beginning to show that consistent yoga practice can reverse osteoporosis and osteopenia. Below is a quote from Dr. Loren Fishman, whose recent pilot study produced the following results.

"Evidence in the animal literature confirms that unconventional tugs of the sinews and ligaments can not only arrest, but reverse osteoporosis. In a pilot study we compared twelve people who completed two years of yoga (the intervention group) with seven people that did not do yoga, the controls. These people had the same average age (66 years), very nearly the same amount of bone loss when the study started, and all had normal laboratory values. By doing 10-12 minutes of yoga a day, the mean bone mineral density of all the patients has improved well beyond that of the controls." (The study can be downloaded at: **sciatica.org/downloads/YogaOsteoporosis_PilotStudy.pdf**)

> *Unconventional tugs of the sinews and ligaments can not only arrest, but reverse osteoporosis.*
> *— Dr. Loren Fishman*

Allow me to offer a personal testimony to the bone-strengthening power of yoga. In the autumn of 2012, at the age of 60, I was working on a ladder that stood on a landing above three brick steps. The grass I'd walked across to my work location was wet and the soles of my shoes were slicker than a banana peel. As I mounted the second step on the ladder, my foot slipped inside the ladder's structure and down I went, falling more than six feet to the bricks below. I landed squarely on my hip joint. After a co-worker graciously cleaned and bandaged multiple abrasions, I went back to a full day of work. I did have a nasty, colorful contusion on my hip, but made a complete and rapid recovery. My years of yoga practice had helped me protect the durability of my femur and hip joint, bones commonly affected by fractures in middle and old age.

This instructive little story brings us to the subject of balance. What are the components of balance? Anyone who has tried to stand on one leg can tell you, you must be strong to hold your balance, and you must concentrate on the act of balancing. Balance, as I tell my students, is a function of strength and focus.

The poses contained in *The Dynamic Dozen* offer you an efficient and accessible way to strengthen your muscles, balance, and bones. I've chosen these particular poses for their effectiveness and because they are easy for the novice yoga student to perform.

Hatha Yoga is not a miracle cure, a religion, or a mystifying esoteric practice that only a select few can understand. It is a practical system of breathing and movement that anyone can learn. As one of Hatha Yoga's great contemporary teachers, B.K.S. Iyengar, proclaimed, "Yoga is universal culture." Anyone can practice Hatha Yoga and gain its many benefits.

> *I call yoga the "universal tool box." Any question about health can be addressed by some facet of yoga.*

A myth about Hatha Yoga that must be immediately dispelled is that you have to be flexible to participate. Even those with a limited range of motion and strength or with advanced disease can begin a Hatha Yoga practice. It is so adaptable that, after twenty years of personal practice and teaching, I call yoga the "universal tool box." Any question about health can be addressed by some facet of yoga.

But the issues at hand are bone density, balance, and your ability to live independently. In *The Dynamic Dozen*, you will learn to use the tools and gain the skills of Hatha Yoga to begin building bone density and balance today.

How the Poses Work

By now you might well ask, "How can practicing these funny-looking poses help rebuild my bone density?" **The answer is resistance to gravity.** As we place our bodies into various positions to counter gravity, our bones respond to the exertion of bearing weight by growing more bone cells from the nutrients in our food. It is a simple, elegant, natural process.

Hatha Yoga, because of the variety of ingenious postures, has extraordinary power to help you rebuild bone density. These poses are low-impact and can be modified to suit your level of health and fitness.

By practicing the postures you see in these pages a few minutes per day, three to five days per week, you will likely be able to return to normal healthy bone density and increase your balance at the same time. If your schedule is demanding, you could practice four postures a day and rotate your poses in a three-day cycle. Regular, persistent, enjoyable practice will help you reach your goal of strong bones, balance, and a confident, independent life-style.

How to Begin

First, choose a pleasant room in your home or a nice, level, shady spot outdoors for your practice space. Next, buy a yoga mat that gives good traction for your hands and bare feet. Yoga mats can be easily purchased at sporting goods stores, big box retailers, or online at Hugger Mugger (huggermugger.com) or Gaiam (gaiam.com).

Remove your shoes and socks and sit comfortably on your mat in an easy cross-legged pose or a chair if it's more comfortable. Push the sitting bones down and lift the chest and abdomen long into an erect but relaxed posture. (The sitting bones, or the ischial tuberosities, are the bones of the posterior pelvis that are cushioned by the muscles of the buttocks.) Row the shoulders up and back to assure that the chest is open. It is much easier for the heart and lungs to work when the shoulders and chest are open and relaxed. A slouching, concave chest and shoulders put more pressure on the heart and lungs and lend themselves to poor breathing habits that deprive the body of oxygen.

The Breath

Learning to use the full capacity of your lungs is essential to your practice of Hatha Yoga. We'll begin by learning the basic **three-part yoga breath**. This breath is likely a fuller breath than you are accustomed to taking. That does not mean you have to use a lot of effort to practice this technique. Never strain yourself beyond your capacity when practicing Hatha Yoga. My motto is: Gentleness is the path to strength. Strain and over-exertion lead to injury. Mindful, gentle practice leads to strength, greater awareness, and abundant health.

> *Gentleness is the path to strength. Strain and over-exertion lead to injury. Mindful, gentle practice leads to strength, greater awareness, and abundant health.*

The next time you're able to observe a child sleeping, notice how the belly rises and falls with the inhalation and exhalation. This is the natural, instinctive way our breath is supposed to work. In order to look svelte and trim, some of us have gotten into the habit of holding in our abdomens which prevents air from fully inflating the lower lobes of our lungs. By doing so, we exchange our natural abdominal breathing rhythm for chest breathing that pulls the abdomen in rather than pushing it out. When the bottom lobes of the lungs are not fully expanded, this deprives the abdominal organs of the therapeutic massage of a normal breath. If, as you inhale, you suck your abdomen in, you may well be creating subtle, chronic tension in your body.

Part 1. To fully oxygenate the body, we must completely utilize the lungs—bottom, middle, and top. Place one hand on your belly, below your waist. Breathe into the belly only. It should swell with the inhalation and fall with the exhalation. (If your belly falls on the inhalation, you are reverse-breathing. Start again, until the first part of the breath feels natural to you.) Continue breathing into the belly for several more breaths until it becomes comfortable and natural.

Part 2. Now place the other hand on the middle of your torso, the area known as your solar plexus. As you find the belly filling up with breath, draw the breath up into the ribs so that you are now doing a two-part breath. Feel the ribs spread out as the rising breath pushes up into the middle of your torso. The diaphragm is the lateral sheet of muscle that divides the chest and abdomen. Notice how the descending diaphragm gently massages the solar plexus.

> *Conscious, controlled breathing can help us control our emotions and can be a life-saver in emergency situations.*

Part 3. Lastly, as the breath moves up from the belly into the mid torso, continue inhaling as you pull it up through the chest and under the collar bones to complete the three-part breath. Remember that although this is a much deeper breath than you usually take, it should still be easy and practically effortless with NO straining. You're not trying to inhale the entire atmosphere of the planet, just a nice, full, rejuvenating breath.

The conscious use of the breath can have tremendous benefits. As we perform Hatha Yoga postures, the breath acts as your own personal massage therapist. As you begin your practice you will feel how the breath reaches into your muscles, organs, and glands to massage and tone them.

Conscious, controlled breathing can also help us control our emotions and can be a life-saver in emergency situations. For example, at 50, Hunter is the picture of vibrant health and loves her yoga practice. During a holiday with her family she was riding a Segway, the two-wheeled personal transport device. She crashed, severely spraining her ankle and back. In moments Hunter found herself alone in an emergency department treatment room waiting for a doctor. She felt herself going into shock. She desperately wanted to do something to help herself. She remembered the simple three-part breath we'd practiced so many times in yoga class. As she focused and breathed consciously she blocked the advance of shock and restored herself to calm, lucid, normal awareness. Hunter realized the potential of her breath and felt empowered because she was able to help herself in a moment of critical need.

Another student, Debbie, had an inspirational experience one night when she awoke in panic to the onset of an asthma attack. She'd been taking my class weekly at her work place. As her fear of the attack grew, she suddenly remembered our three-part breathing practice in class. She began to take slow, deep, conscious breaths, which dampened her fear and allowed her to address this emergency with calm control. In a matter of seconds she was able to quell her asthma attack and enjoy a restful night's sleep just by remembering her breath. So, if you've never thought about breathing as a powerful way to heal—think again.

A Note on Your Breathing

If, at any time, your breath becomes ragged or uneven as you practice, reduce your effort or come out of the pose and rest. A disturbed breathing pattern is a sure sign that you are either trying too hard or you are not ready for the pose you are attempting.

The Sigh

As another way to use the breath, I heartily recommend sighing to help release tension after the exertion of any pose. Despite our best efforts we often try too hard to perform a yoga pose. This excess effort can build tension in our bodies. Sighing is not merely a by-product of yawning, laughter, or sex. Sighing is a multi-purpose breathing technique that releases physical as well as emotional tension. Through physical or mental exertion, tension builds up in our bodies. Sighing encourages deep abdominal breathing that massages tension away. A long, slow exhalation encourages relaxation. Try it and you will see a definite difference in how you feel. My students know me as a rather noisy yogi because of my propensity to use this marvelous natural technique for stress relief.

Comfortable Engagement Yoga

A word about intensity and effort in your practice

In our competitive culture even yoga has become contaminated by the attitude of struggle and strain. In yoga studios and sports clubs all over the country, yoga is often reduced to little more than a glorified callisthenic.

The word *yoga* comes from the ancient Sanskrit root *yug*, meaning to yoke or unify. Yoga is about the union of body, mind, and soul with the great universal creative consciousness, call it whatever you will. The second century B.C. sage Patanjali defined yoga as the ability to focus the mind on one thing to the exclusion of all others. Rather than being just the latest workout craze, yoga is both a spiritual and a physical art and science.

As you practice, apply enough effort to feel engaged in the pose, but not so much that you cannot readily smile. If your face and body are tense because of the effort you are pouring into your practice, you are working too hard. I teach a style of practice that I call **comfortable engagement yoga**.

> *Yoga is the ability to focus the mind on one thing to the exclusion of all others.*
> – *Patanjali*
> 2nd century B.C. sage

Once you have assumed the basic architecture of any pose, the breath is applied generously to open the body completely and safely. Allow the breath and your comfortably engaged pose to take you to a state of bliss within your activity. Never should you strain to get your posture "perfect." There is no striving for perfection in yoga, just joyful practice as you create many magical moments of serendipity. Be grateful for those moments. They will be more abundant when you practice with gentleness, attention, and gratitude. The "no pain, no gain" attitude has no place in yoga.

Remember, gentleness is the path to strength. With that as your affirmation, you enable yourself to practice with safety and enjoyment.

The Rest

As you work your way through the poses, feel free to rest between postures for a few breaths at any time. This is not an endurance contest, so don't feel as if you have to push through this series of poses just because you think you should. Lie down after every pose if you like. Take some nice, easy, full breaths. Then allow the breath to return to normal for a thorough restorative rest. Listen to your body!

You're doing something new, so give yourself a break and rest as you work your way through the poses. Use your three-part breath and a sigh after each one to encourage full-body relaxation. That way you can begin the next pose feeling rejuvenated and calm.

The Poses

Though there are many great yoga poses to address the myriad aspects of preventing and healing disease, I've chosen what I call *The Dynamic Dozen* to help you rebuild your bone density and balance. These poses each have one thing in common: **They use simple structural shapes to put your body into various relationships to gravity that will stimulate your body to start making bone cells.** You will feel the power of this yoga architecture when you practice poses like warrior, triangle, bridge, and bow.

Additionally, these postures encourage circulation in a way that no other form of movement can. As we bend forward, backward, and to the side, gravity helps pull the blood flow throughout the body. This is why children are so supple. As they play, they are constantly moving their bodies into ever-changing orientations to gravity. As we grow we assume what I call the three primary adult postures: standing, sitting, and lying. That's when our strength, balance, and range of motion begin to decline. Our yoga postures help us to wash away the years and restore our flexibility, strength, and range of motion.

When you look at *The Dynamic Dozen* poses, they may not look very aerobic. Sustaining the postures for several breaths, however, will increase your heart and respiration rates. Check your heart rate after some of these poses and you'll see what I mean. Yoga works the whole body gently and thoroughly.

Each posture has its own shape or architecture. This architecture can either be passive or active. Just because we have assumed the basic shape of the pose doesn't mean we are actively engaged in it. Active, comfortable engagement means using the complementary forces of pushing and pulling, grounding and reaching.

> *Active, comfortable engagement means using the complementary forces of pushing and pulling, grounding and reaching*

For example, the standing poses always involve grounding the feet into the earth or floor. From the waist down, the legs are active and we feel a sense of rootedness. From the waist up, we are either reaching up, as in Warrior I, or reaching out, as in Warrior II. We use the complementary forces of gravity and levity, or lightness. By activating these complementary opposites we engage the whole body in the pose.

From there we can find a state of repose and calm in the midst of our activity. This is done by using the three-part breath to make each pose a meditation as well as a bone-density and balance-building activity. In this way we engage both the active and restful parts (sympathetic and parasympathetic) of our nervous systems simultaneously. This is why we feel both invigorated and calm after our practice.

How About Weights?

You might wonder, could I use weights instead? Yes, you could, but I would argue that they are neither as safe nor effective as yoga postures. There are no weight machines that mimic the way yoga poses stimulate the healing response from head to toe. Weights and weight machines isolate various body parts for a particular motion. Though there is nothing wrong with that in and of itself, using weights cannot integrate motion and breath to engage the whole body at one time the way yoga postures do. Also, yoga postures use the weight of your own body, with which you are intimately familiar. There is no guessing about how much weight to use and no risk of misjudging that amount, a misjudgment that could lead to injury. This is especially helpful if you're already dealing with bones that may be near the fracture threshold.

The Standing Poses

Mountain

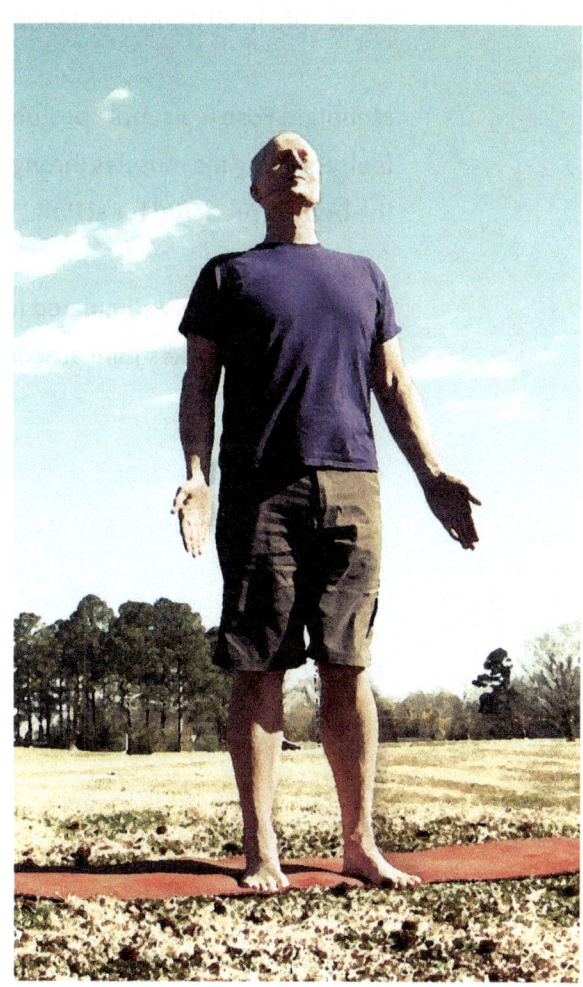

Basic mountain pose is a simple and easy place to begin. **Stand with the feet directly below the hips, the chest and heart open, and the breath smooth and full.** ■ **Lengthen the torso and spine** as you firmly push the feet into the ground. Feel the muscles of the legs engage as you root yourself into the earth with confidence and stability. ■ **Draw the knee caps up** to activate the muscles in the front of your thighs. ■ **Stand and breathe.** Sense the crown of your head reaching skyward as your torso lengthens. Feel the firm but relaxed muscular engagement of your entire body. Imagine you are a mountain with all the strength and solidity that your mental picture implies.

The Benefits

As we practice Mountain Pose or any other pose, we unify our physical posture with our mental posture. Remember, yoga means union. So rather than just performing a physical posture like posing for a picture, we want to completely embody the physicality of our yoga by inviting our minds and emotions into the willful act of establishing ourselves in our practice.

Mountain

Mountain Pose is the beginning of learning to concentrate, of building focus as we engage in the physical act of Hatha Yoga. It gives us the foundational attitude for the rest of our practice. We develop the feeling of being immovable and centered in the Earth. If you enjoy visualization, take your "mountainhood" as far as you want to go. See yourself being thrust up from the earth to harbor life in all its manifestations.

Mountain Pose is a simple posture that teaches us to engage our whole body. As we ground our feet, engaging the muscles throughout our torso and arms, we are conscious of how each part of the body is prepared for action.

The joints are gently stimulated to produce synovial fluid, the juicy liquid that provides the **slide and glide** that makes joint articulation so effortless.

Warrior II

The warrior poses have nothing to do with war or violence. For me, they are about developing an attitude of strength, sense of place, and self-mastery.

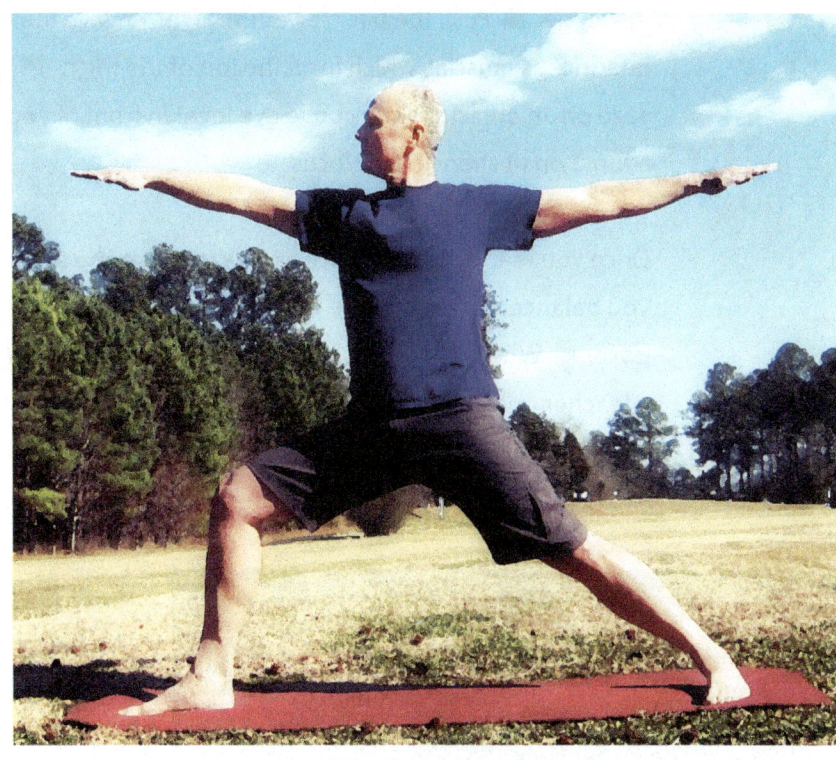

If your balance is not reliable, practice near a wall or a sturdy chair so you can catch yourself should you get a little wobbly. Otherwise, your practice space should be free and clear of obstructions. ■ Begin in **Mountain Pose**. Push the feet gently into the ground, be long through the torso and bring the hands to the heart in gratitude and awareness of the powerful practice in which you are about to participate. Remember, millions of people presently and throughout history have walked the path that you are now beginning. Use that thought to inspire your practice. ■ **Walk your feet to a parallel stance** about three feet apart, perhaps a bit more if you have long legs. We are working with stability in mind here, so be conservative and safe. ■ **Turn the right foot out** 90 degrees forward and the left foot 45 to 90 degrees inward as pictured. The torso is stacked directly above the pelvis, so that you sense your spine rising from its base.

The toes are relaxed at all times and the soles are firmly grounded by pushing the feet into the ground. If you're not using a mat and find your carpet or flooring slippery, put on some shoes

Warrior II

with a non-skid sole. ■ **Bend the right knee** anywhere from just slightly bent to the point that your shin and thigh form a 90-degree angle. Make sure the knee is aligned directly above the ankle. ■ Push the back leg out straight, engage the tendon below the kneecap and the big quadriceps muscles which form the top of the thigh. ■ Get your balance and feel stable. Fix your gaze on an object slightly above eye level in front of you for a focus point. Remember, balance is a function of strength and focus.

Once you feel steady in stance and gaze, **raise the arms** out to an airplane configuration to help you balance like a tight rope walker. ■ Take a couple of breaths here to get accustomed to the pose. ■ When you feel balanced **shift the right arm forward and the left arm back**. I heard a teacher once say that the backward reaching arm is in the past, the front arm is reaching into the future, and the mind and heart are in the present. I like the integration of past, present, and future in this description.

> *Below the waist we are grounded, above the waist we are reaching. This is the simultaneous expression of gravity and levity.*

This is the basic architecture of the pose. To energize the posture, push down into the feet and legs as you reach up from the waist and through the shoulders and arms. Below the waist we are grounded, above the waist we are reaching. We push into the earth with the feet and legs and reach up to the heavens with our torso, arms, and gaze. This is the simultaneous expression of gravity and levity.

Feel all the muscles in the respective regions of the body respond with firmness and activity. Pay special attention to the **quadriceps** (the big muscles above the kneecap), the **hamstrings** (beneath the thigh bone), and the **gluteus muscles** of the buttocks. Recruit all these muscles simultaneously to support this pose. ■ Now activate the full, easy, **three-part breath**. Keep your focus and your sense of groundedness as you practice Warrior II. As you breathe feel how

Warrior II

the distance between the feet makes you work to sustain this pose. ■ As the feet push firmly in opposite directions, the leg bones and muscles are fully engaged. Continue to breathe deeply and smoothly with your three-part breath. ■ **Visualize and feel how the breath massages** the entire body, and how the lungs and heart are pumping high volumes of freshly oxygenated blood throughout your body.

Be steady and strong as you hold the pose. Even though you are exerting yourself, breathe your way into a relaxed exertion. Remember, if you are trying so hard that you can't smile, you're working too hard. Ease up a bit and enjoy yourself. **Be comfortably engaged** in your body while you hold this wonderfully effective pose. ■ As you begin to feel fatigue slowly lower the arms and bring the feet parallel and step back into Mountain Pose and relax. ■ After a few relaxing recovery breaths, **practice the pose on the other side**. As you practice on the opposite side, notice whether the pose seems easier or more difficult. Yoga will always show us if we have any asymmetries in our bodies, and it will help us to correct those imbalances with gentle, persistent practice.

> *As always, come out of a pose when you feel you must, but also be willing to challenge yourself a little bit every time you practice.*

I've watched my beginning students with osteoporosis in the standing poses. They sometimes groan when I encourage them to hold the poses a little longer to build endurance. Their legs may quiver with weakness, but after consistent practice their strength increases along with their balance and confidence. Feel free to support yourself with a wall or chair if necessary. As always, come out of a pose when you feel you must, but also be willing to challenge yourself a little bit every time you practice.

Warrior II

The Benefits

The quadriceps, gluteus muscles, and hamstrings are all strengthened by the warrior poses, along with the tendons and ligaments throughout the legs. The adductor muscles on the inside of the thighs are also toned and strengthened. The knees, hips, and ankles gain great endurance from these poses. Consistent practice of Warrior II will begin the process of building denser bones and better balance.

Warrior I

Warrior I is similar to its sister pose, Warrior II, but with some subtle, important distinctions.

Beginning again in **Mountain Pose**, step the feet out into the standard wide stance with the feet parallel. ■ Turn the right foot out to 90 degrees and the left foot to 45 to 90 degrees, as with Warrior II.

Here's where the pose changes. Turn the torso so that it is pointing in the same direction as the front (right) leg. The right big toe, knee, hip, right ribs and the sternoclavicular joint (the joint created by the top of the breast bone and the collar bone) should all be aligned. There may be a tendency for the torso to rotate a bit toward the back leg, so keep your alignment in mind as you practice this pose.

Once you feel stable, lift the arms slowly upward. If balance is a problem, try airplane arms or simply take the hands to the waist. ■ As in Warrior II, firmly push the feet into the floor, relax the toes, and feel the muscular engagement of the feet and legs. ■ Use the easy, deep, three-part breaths to fully oxygenate and cleanse the body. Hold your pose with attention and focus. Allow nothing to divert your gaze. Practice breathing your way into relaxed exertion, as if the pose were a meditation. In my early days of yoga practice I heard it said that yoga is a meditation and each posture is a prayer. Though I'm not a religious

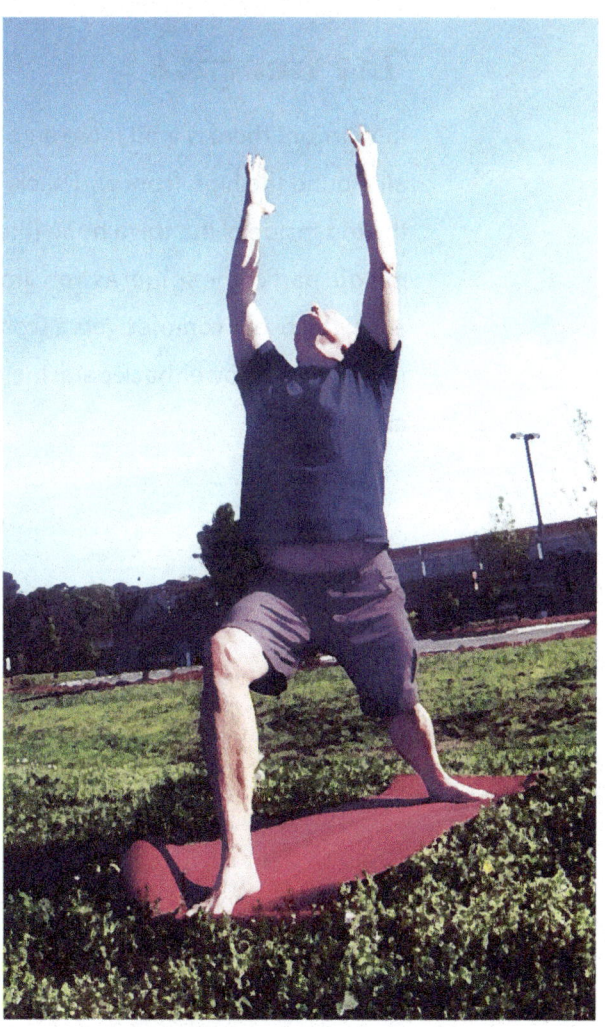

19

Warrior I

person, I still like to think of yoga in those terms. ■ As you are prompted by your body to come out of the posture, **return to Mountain Pose** ■ Practice Warrior I on the other side.

The Benefits

In Warrior I there is a bit more emphasis on strengthening the muscles in the lower abdomen and all around the hips, front and back. The muscles known as psoas major and psoas minor connect the top inside of the thigh bone (the femur), through the pelvis, and up to the vertebrae of the middle part of the spine. As you ground your feet and legs and reach up through the torso and arms, the psoas complex gets a wonderful stretch and toning. Weak psoas muscles can contribute to chronic lower back pain. Incidentally, the psoas is the fillet mignon cut of beef in bovine anatomy.

Tree

This is a pure balance pose because all the weight of the body is borne on one leg. In my classes I often mention the bristlecone pine tree or the majestic sequoia when we prepare for this pose. For me, this pose represents understanding who you are, your sense of place, and your rootedness in that place. The bristlecone and the sequoia live rooted to one spot for thousands of years. I like to try to imagine that deep, mysterious sense of place when I practice this pose. Give it a try!

If you need to practice near the wall to help you stay in the pose, by all means do it. This pose may challenge your sense of balance like no other.

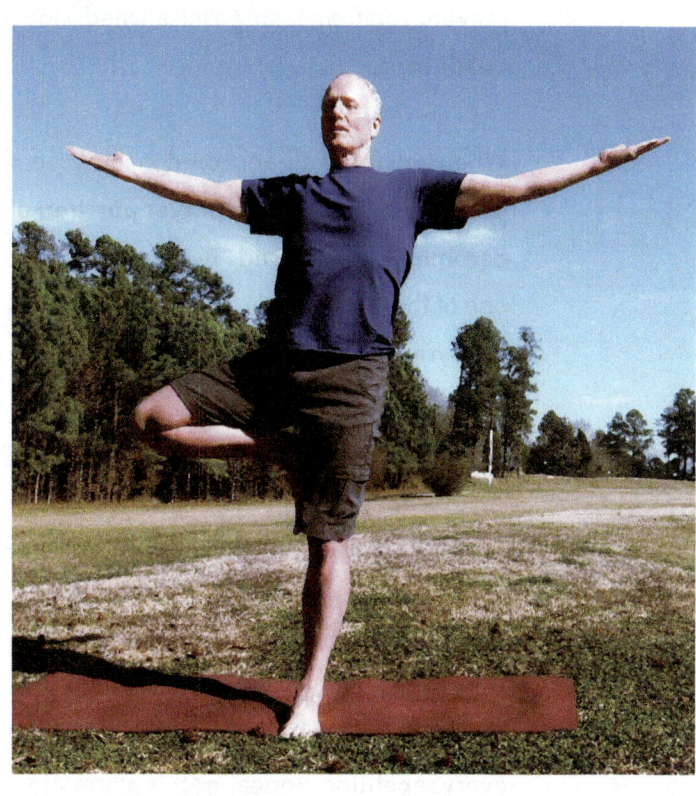

Stand in **Mountain Pose** with the feet equally grounded, the legs active and engaged, and the breath smooth. ■ Slowly lift one leg with the sole of that foot sliding up the inside of the grounded leg. Use your hand to help place the foot in the desired position above the knee if you can. ■ **Press the sole of the foot into the standing leg** to keep it in position. ■ Breathe and focus to stabilize yourself. ■ If that's too difficult, then positioning your foot at the shin or ankle are fine, too. The purpose of the pose is to strengthen the muscles and bones, not achieve a "pretty" or ideal pose. Your form will improve with practice. ■ Fix your gaze somewhere on the floor.

Tree

Avoid placing the foot against the knee. The knee is a hinge joint. Its lateral movement is practically nonexistent. ■ **Push firmly into the grounded leg** so the hip joint is active. This will prevent you from taking a misaligned, slouching posture. ■ **Draw the kneecap up** to engage the quadriceps.

When you feel well-anchored in the pose, **slowly extend the arms out and up like an airplane, or bring them to prayer position at the heart**. ■ Remain here, breathing deeply as you become more balanced. ■ You may then raise your arms above the head and imagine you are one of the great, sturdy, immovable trees I spoke about earlier. Go inward as you breathe and hold your gaze. Enjoy this rooted, solid, abiding Tree Pose.

Repeat this affirmation: I am getting stronger every time I practice.

Listen to your ankle because it will start talking to you. Feel it moving in its internal dance as it works to keep you in the pose. ■ **Keep breathing** and hold the pose until the ankle begins to feel fatigue. ■ Slowly allow your bent leg to return to the floor and rest in Mountain Pose. ■ Now **practice the pose on the other side**.

If you lose your balance, rest for a few breaths and try the pose again. You will get stronger with every repetition. Repeating this affirmation with commitment will help you with Tree Pose or any other: I am getting stronger every time I practice.

The Benefits

All the leg joints are strengthened, especially the ankle. Concentration and mental acuity are also sharpened as you hone your focus to maintain the pose. Tree Pose builds perseverance and strong character. When you lose your balance, try again. Your persistence will be rewarded without a doubt. Best of all, the one-legged balance poses are superior weight-bearing messengers that tell the body to build bone density.

Dancer's Pose

This beautiful pose will certainly leave you feeling invigorated. ■ Begin again in Mountain Pose. Take expansive, even breaths, with the gaze focused in front of you on the ground nearby. ■ **Slowly lift the right leg**, bending the knee behind you. ■ **Catch the foot** with the right hand. ■ **Draw the knee cap up** on the left leg to engage the quadriceps on the front of the thigh. If you need help with your balance, face the wall and reach out in front of you. ■ This is the first stage of the pose. If proceeding to the following stages is too difficult, be content to remain in this first stage until you build the strength and balance to proceed. ■ **Breathe deeply** into your three-part breath, **push down** into the grounded foot and enjoy.

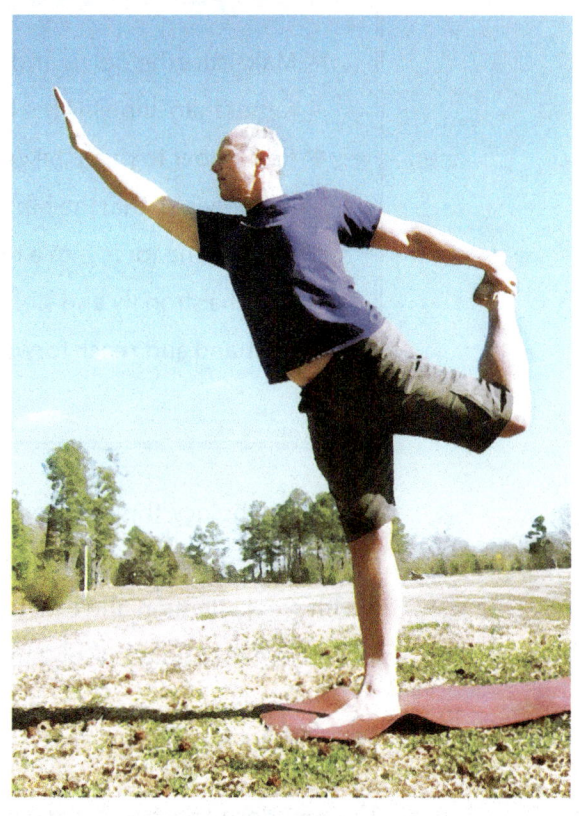

Be patient, begin where you are, and respect your body's current capabilities.

Once you've developed stability in the first stage of Dancer's Pose, **push the right foot into the hand**. This will engage the right shoulder and move the spine into a broad, taut arc. ■ When you are ready, proceed by **lifting the left arm up**. Feel how this accentuates the arc in the spine as the chest swells forward. If you are using the wall, depend upon it as little as possible. ■ Once you've gained your balance with the help of the wall, **begin incrementally reducing your contact with it** so that your body becomes more active in the pose. Depending on your fitness, this may take awhile. Be patient, begin where you are, and respect your body's current capabilities. Delight in the massaging quality of the breath. ■ Repeat on the other side.

Dancer's Pose

> ### Tips for Dancer's Pose
>
> * Make sure the pelvis and lifted leg are still squarely facing the ground rather than allowing the hip to flare open to the side.
> * Remember to push the grounded leg into the earth and lift up through the pelvis so that the hip joint is alive with activity and length as you breathe the torso into a refreshing bow shape.
> * Breathe strongly and steadily as you keep pushing the lifted foot into the hand and reach forward and up with the outstretched hand.

In yoga mythology, this is the pose of the cosmic dancer, dancing creation into existence. Dancer's Pose is one of the most demanding standing poses in this Dynamic Dozen series. Approach it with great attention and care to build your balance and endurance slowly. Before long, you will feel the creative potential of Dancer's Pose.

The Benefits

This wonderful posture builds strength in the legs, opens the chest, and gives the spine gentle, gravity-resisting compression. Dancer's Pose also massages the kidneys and adrenal glands. The one-legged poses build extraordinary physical balance, strength, and mental concentration and provide superior gravity resistance to build bone density.

Remember, even though the one-legged poses are difficult, they are central to building bone density. Practice them with whole-hearted enthusiasm. As you practice Dancer's Pose you may begin to feel an expansive, all-embracing attitude towards life.

Warrior III

I must confess that as I began to practice Warrior III many years ago, it was not an instant favorite. In fact, I rather avoided it. It was hard, and like many difficult things, it was easy to justify my avoidance and allow that part of my body to remain undeveloped. One day I accepted the challenge of Warrior III. My strength, balance, and confidence have all increased since I embraced this pose. It's one of my favorite poses now, and one that will be of great benefit in protecting and rebuilding your bone density.

If, when you first try Warrior III, you find yourself reacting as I did, be courageous and ready to begin an intimate friendship with this powerful pose. Take the pose in small doses at first, building your strength mindfully. Soon you will experience the wonderful rewards of balance, strength, and stronger bones.

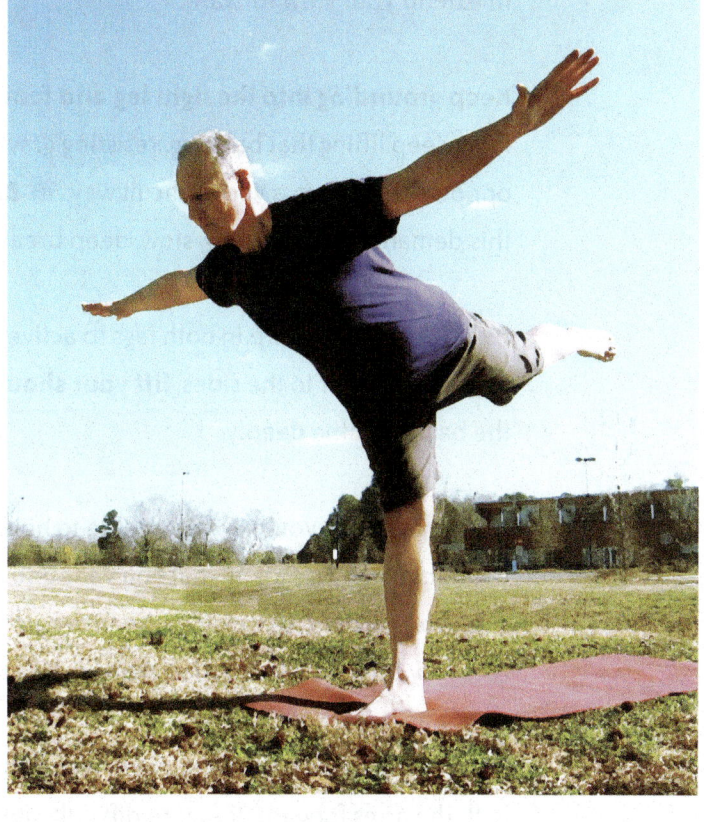

Stand in Mountain Pose with the feet firmly grounded and begin with the three-part conscious breath. ■ When you feel ready, remain grounded in the right foot, **extend your hands either behind you or to your sides like an airplane for balance**. When you're ready to challenge yourself a bit more, reach your arms forward. ■ **Slowly begin to bend forward at the hip** and raise the left leg off the ground behind you. Raise the lifted leg as high as you comfortably can. Ideally, the lifted leg, torso and head should be aligned at the same level. This may take a while.

Warrior III

Enjoy the challenge and be persistent. ■ **Focus your gaze on some spot on the floor** to help you concentrate. Fix your gaze directly below you to begin with. As you gain mastery in Warrior III extend your view forward.

Keep grounding into the right leg and foot so that the hip joint of the standing leg is active and long. Keep lifting that back leg, resisting gravity. This will take a bit of effort. Most of your body is opposing gravity in a very difficult way. ■ **Breathe deeply** to feed your body lots of oxygen for this demanding pose. Long, slow, deep breaths will help you sustain Warrior III.

Pull the knee caps up in both legs to active the quadriceps. ■ As you extend your arms either in back of you or to the sides, **lift your shoulders and chest upward** and feel the natural arch of the back. Breathe deeply.

In the beginning you may not be able to hold the pose very long, but that's to be expected. Accept your ability and be joyful that you've found one of the jewels of the Dynamic Dozen. ■ **Slowly release Warrior III** as your endurance wanes and return to Mountain Pose. Take a few restful recovery breaths. ■ **Practice Warrior III on the other side**.

When you've gained some strength and mastery in this posture, Warrior III may be practiced with the arms forward. It's more difficult, but extending the arms will help you develop greater strength in your shoulders and arms, along with a victorious attitude.

The Benefits

Warrior III builds exceptional strength and balance. The muscles of the back, legs, and buttocks really get a great work out. This pose also stabilizes all the joints in the legs, especially the knee. As with the other one-legged balance poses, Warrior III develops superior balance, concentration, and strong bones.

Triangle

If balance is challenging for you, you can practice Triangle Pose with your back close to a clear wall. ■ Start in **Mountain Pose**. ■ **Step the legs out** to the side as you did in Warrior I and II. The feet are parallel. ■ **Rotate the right foot out 90 degrees** and position the **back foot between 45 and 90 degrees**. ■ Place the right hand above the right knee and place the left hand on the left hip. ■ **Sweep the left arm up** and roll the chest toward the left shoulder so that the entire torso is open. ■ Inhale a centering three-part breath.

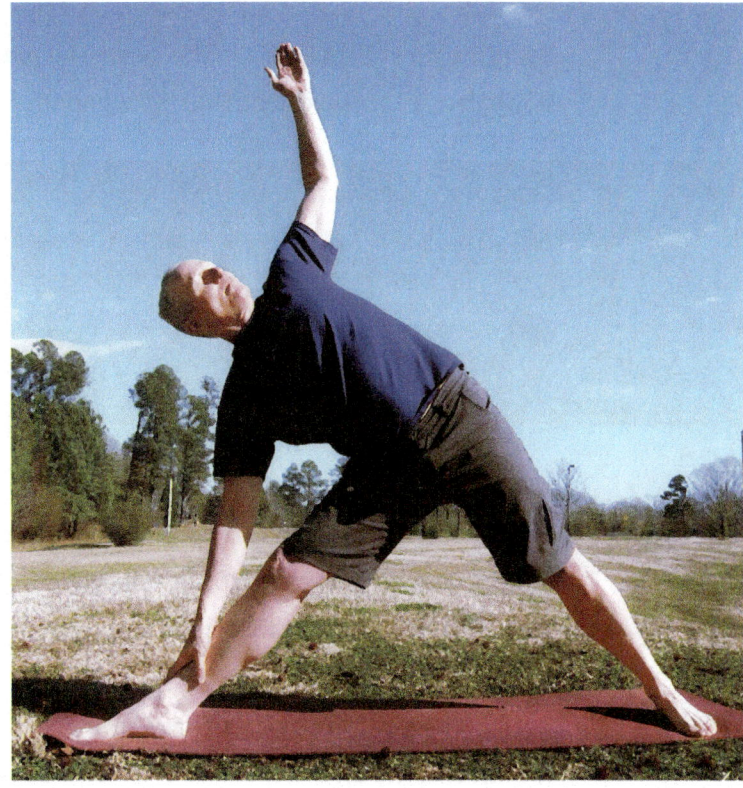

Now, **slowly slide the right hand down the shin bone** until it's somewhere between your knee and your ankle. The farther down you slide the hand, the greater stretch you'll get in your hamstrings, back of the knee, and calf. Your hand may be just below your knee to begin with. The point is to be comfortable, at ease, and aware of how you feel in the pose. One of my favorite yoga quotes comes from yogi Max Strom. Max says, "Remember, it doesn't matter how deep into a posture you go—what does matter is who you are when you get there."

If your left shoulder begins to curl toward the ground as the right hand descends, stop there and rise until the chest is once again open and the left arm is pointing straight up. Try to keep the

Triangle

body in a flat plane, as if flattened against a wall. You'll reap more benefit from extending into this plane than from letting your shoulder be drawn down toward the ground.

Using the wall will help you in this pose. **You may certainly lean into the wall** to help you stay balanced as you extend into the wonderful stretch provided by Triangle Pose. Once you've developed more strength, you can be less dependent on the wall.

"Remember, it doesn't matter how deep into a posture you go—what does matter is who you are when you get there."
—Yogi Max Strom

Firmly push the feet into the ground in opposite directions and press the right hand into the shin bone to stabilize the posture. ■ As you ground your feet, you may notice a subtle inner rotation of the calf muscles of both legs. The grounding of the feet will also pull the buttocks and sacrum into alignment with the spine. This is very important. If the buttocks are hanging out in space, unaligned with the spine, the hamstrings will be unnecessarily strained. Please be mindful of this important alignment of buttocks, sacrum, and spinal column.

Recruit the quadriceps by pulling the kneecap up. This will engage the tendon directly below the knee. ■ **Relax the toes** and ground through the soles of your feet. ■ You may gently turn your head to look up if you like, but it may prove tiring to the neck and may affect your balance. Otherwise, look straight out from the body or look down at the ground to help you balance.

Energize the pose with the full three-part breath. Feel the breath pushing into the hamstrings and other muscles that may be stiff or resistant to this architecture. ■ If the hamstrings feel tight, simply slide the right hand a few inches up the shin for a gentler stretch. As you progress, you will be able to slide the hand farther down the leg without losing the integrity of the open torso. Take your time and enjoy the journey. There is no hurry. ■ As you use just the right amount of exertion to perform this pose, cultivate a restful mental attitude in the midst of your activity.

Triangle

Breathe your way into a comfortably engaged expression of Triangle Pose.

If and when you're ready for a more challenging expression of the pose, **slowly lift the right hand slightly off the leg, bring it to your heart**, and see how much more engagement you get from the core and the spine. Or just rest your fingertips on the shin without leaning on your hand. **The strongest way to practice Triangle Pose with no support from the grounded hand is to reach both arms over your head**. This is a powerful modification of the pose, so approach it with great respect and care. If this modification of Triangle Pose is a bit too demanding, no worries. The standard pose will serve you quite well.

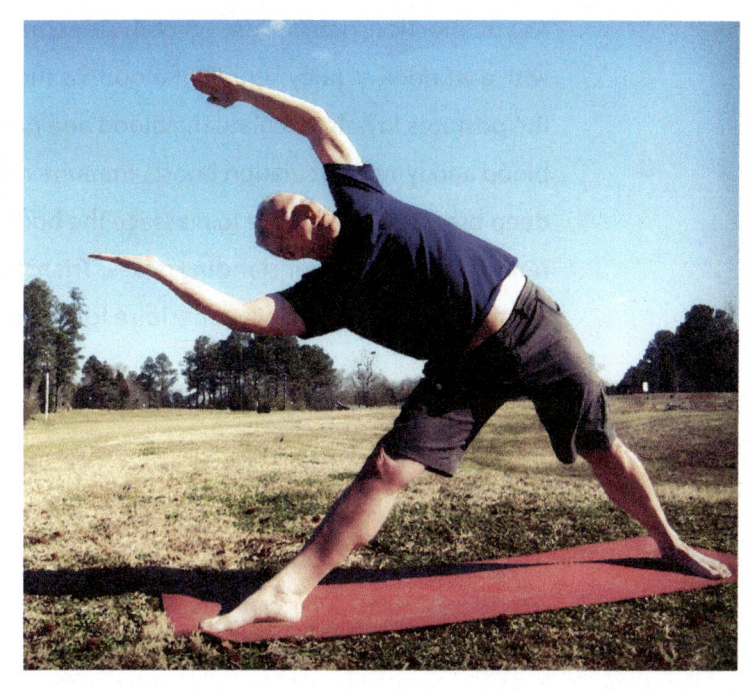

A powerful modification of the pose is to reach both arms out in front of you.

When you're ready, slowly bend the right knee and rise out of the posture and return to Mountain Pose. Feel how the blood pressure changes in the head as you elevate your upper body. ■ **Repeat Triangle Pose on the other side**.

The Benefits

As with all the other poses where the legs are spread wide, you can feel how Triangle Pose builds strong legs and balance. As there is more than just a bit of a spinal twist in this posture, the hip joints, sacroiliac joints and the musculature in the pelvis are thoroughly engaged and toned. The disks and vertebrae also get a good rotation to help keep the back supple.

Triangle

As you practice Triangle Pose on both sides, notice how each hemisphere of the brain is bathed with a wonderful, juicy supply of blood. As the ancient yogis realized, gravity is harnessed by the postures to help circulate the blood and provide lymphatic drainage as well. Increased blood and lymph circulation boosts immune response and organ/gland function. Movement and deep breathing both serve to massage the body, which facilitates nutrient absorption and waste removal. Like the other standing poses, Triangle Pose's wide stance adds another unique weight-bearing shape to your yoga repertoire to help build bone density.

The Sitting and Prone Poses

Cobra

Stage I

As you study and practice yoga, you will notice that many postures are named after animals. The ancient yogis were keen observers of nature. They saw how plants and animals expressed energy through their postures. Cobra Pose is a good example of this observational awareness. In Cobra Pose the torso rises off the ground as the spine arches just like the majestic serpent in ancient Indian mythology.

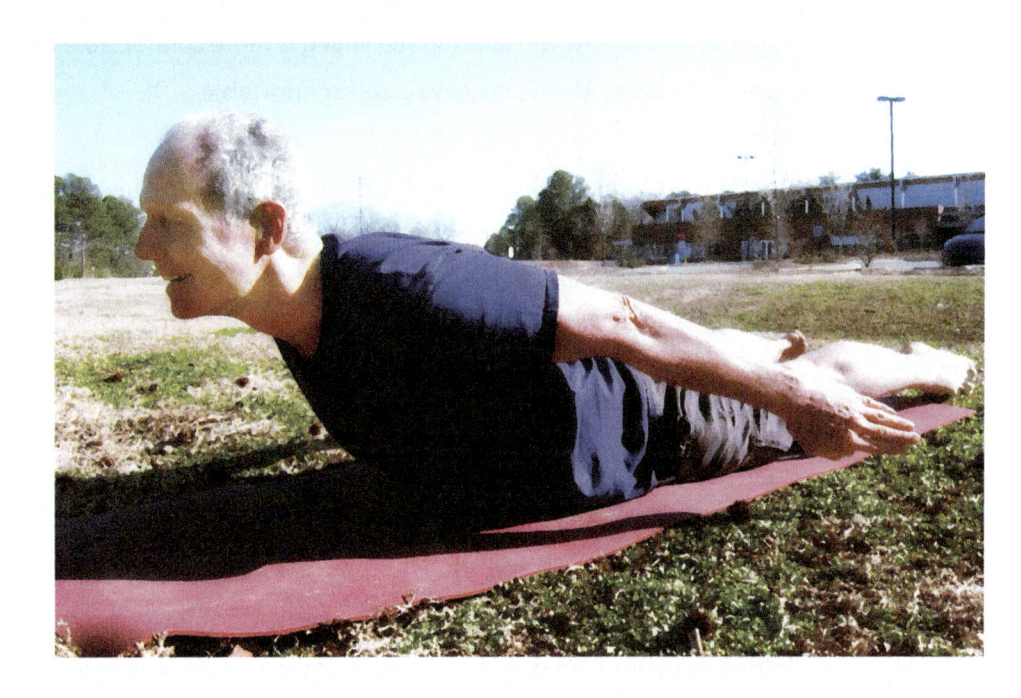

There are several effective ways to practice this simple but powerful pose. In this book, you'll find four variations to practice. I recommend that you sample each of these cobra techniques to find which one you like most. Perhaps a sequence of all of these variations will serve you best. If you attend a yoga class regularly and have a trusted teacher, you could consult them about these variations, too.

Begin by lying down on your belly. Rest your head on folded arms and relax with some nice, gentle, full breaths. Notice the heaviness of your body as you surrender to gravity and relax your

Cobra

weight on the floor. ■ Now, begin with the forehead to the floor, and **on the inhale slowly raise the head, shoulders, and chest** away from the floor by engaging your back and gluteus muscles. ■ As you will in all variations of Cobra Pose, **press the legs firmly into the floor**. Some traditions insist that the feet be together, but I would advise you to try Cobra Pose both ways—feet together and hips-width apart to see which is more comfortable for your body. Remember, your body is the boss. Always make yourself comfortable.

Reach your arms back along each side of your body, palms down. If you need the support of your hands, push the fingertips or palms gently into the floor. You may arch the neck to look up. If this is uncomfortable, simply look straight ahead or down to relieve any strain on the neck.

Breathe deeply and feel how the breath supports this pose. Also, imagine how difficult this pose would be without your abdominal organs. The liver, gall bladder, pancreas, spleen, intestines, stomach, bladder, reproductive organs, and appendix all provide a strong, fluid foundation for Cobra Pose and all of the prone back bends.

Hold the pose to the beginning of fatigue, and then slowly descend and rest your head on your folded arms. Rest, relax, and breathe as you savor the feeling of having engaged your body in a strong gravity-defying way.

Stage II

Rise from your resting posture and extend the arms parallel out in front of you. Make sure your hands are on the mat or ground for maximum

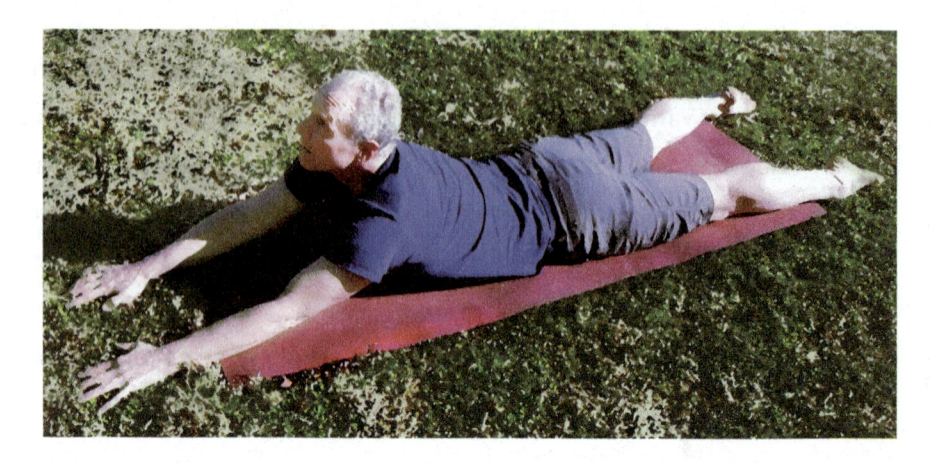

Cobra

traction. Flatten the hands and forearms on the mat. ■ **Ground the hands and forearms and begin to gently pull them back toward your body.** ■ Raise your elbows off the floor. The hands may slide back an inch or two, and that's okay. ■ Simultaneously **reach forward and up with the chest and heart**, so that you are looking out over your hands or, if your neck will allow it, look up for maximum extension. Note the complimentary opposites of pulling grounded hands back and reaching the chest and heart forward. ■ Feel the gentle traction you're getting in the lower portion of your spine. ■ **Breathe gently into the pose**, making any adjustments to maximize your comfort and enjoyment.

I often practice this pose by pulling back with the arms on an inhalation and releasing the pull on the exhalation. Experiment with this technique and enjoy the alternating pull and release timed with your breath. This gives your spine and disks a wonderful massage. ■ **Release the pose** as before and rest the head to the other side. Relax and savor.

Stage III

The next version of Cobra Pose is done with the **elbows directly under the shoulders and the forearms parallel to each other**, palms down so you look like a sphinx. This form of Cobra is often called **Sphinx Pose**.

With the elbows bent and forearms parallel, **ground the hands and forearms, pulling back as you reach forward with the**

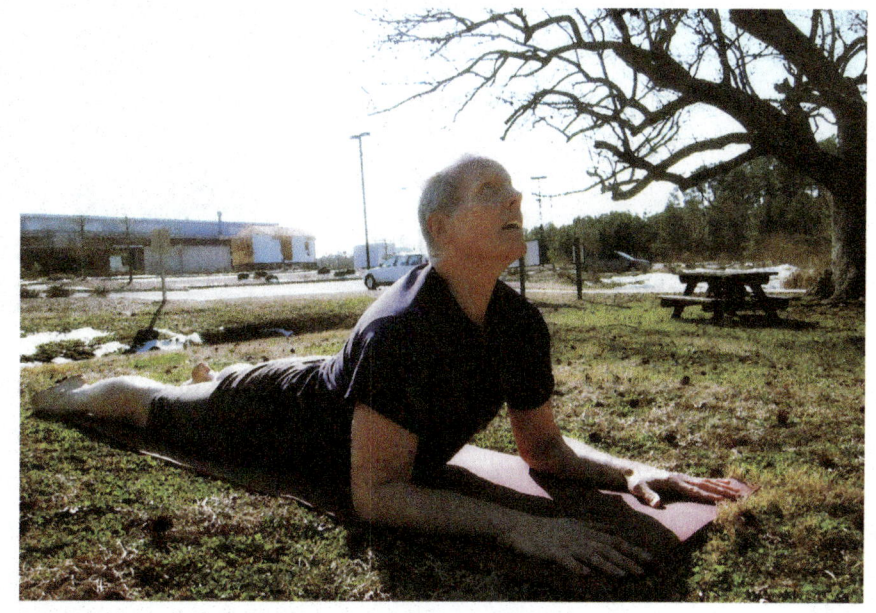

This position is also known as the Sphinx Pose.

Cobra

chest and heart. The reaching and pulling are similar to those in Cobra II, but notice the difference the starting position has made in how the posture feels to you. Since you've moved a bit higher with more of the torso off the ground, the traction you receive as you pull and reach will be a bit more pronounced. Apply your effort consciously and incrementally for optimum results.
■ **Breathe into the pose** and feel the massage of your breath flowing throughout your body. ■ **Listen to your body.** What feels best about the pose? Use that information to make any adjustments you need to enjoy this wonderful back bend. ■ When you're ready, release and slowly come down from the pose and rest.

Stage IV

Remember, gentleness is the path to strength. Of all the ways we've worked with Cobra Pose so far, this is the strongest expression of the posture. Approach it slowly and mindfully.

As you raise the head and chest off the floor slightly, slide the hands back until the finger tips are adjacent to the ribs and nipples. This is a suggestion for the approximate location of your hands. Feel and sense the effect this is having on your body. Find a comfortable position for your hands by experimenting with slightly different placements. ■ **This time, push the hands firmly into the floor** as you also exert a backward pressure. ■ **Reach forward and up** through the torso and feel the same pull and reach as before.

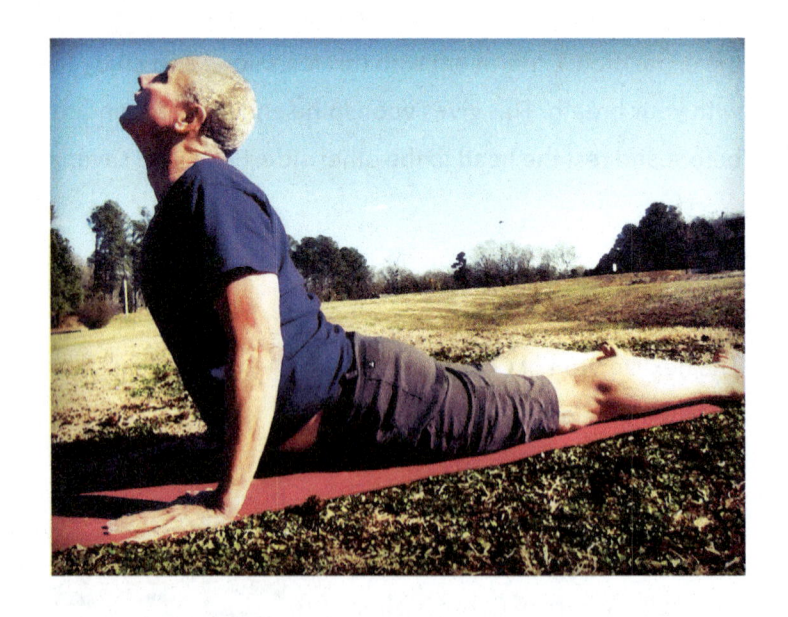

Cobra

This is the point in the practice of Cobra Pose where I see so many students try to overreach. Many beginning students, and even those who have been practicing for a while, think that by pushing their arms straight they are maximizing the effect of the Cobra. Until the back is made supple by repeated practice, this extension may exert too much pressure on the disks.

Keep the elbows bent and hugged close to your body as you exert downward and backward pressure into your hands. ■ As you reach the chest forward you will create a long arc in the back. Straightening the arms before this technique has been mastered often will bend the back at an angle rather than an arc. This can put unnecessary pressure on the vertebrae and disks. Remember, it's not how high you come up in the pose that matters, it's the safe and proper form and shape for the back that is paramount. ■ **Breathe and enjoy the energy moving in your body**. ■ Come out of the pose when you're ready and rest.

If you are a beginning student, I would suggest that you work with Stages I, II, and III for a while before you practice Stage IV. There is no hurry. The first three stages confer the same benefit as the more advanced form. You may notice that you enjoy the first three stages as much or more anyway.

> *Cobra Pose could be called the fountain of youth for the spine.*

I often use one or more of these styles of Cobra Pose in my own practice sessions. Each technique contributes its own unique route to a stronger spine, more elastic disks, and denser bones.

The Benefits

Without exaggeration, Cobra Pose could be called the fountain of youth for the spine. Practicing all the stages of Cobra successively will cultivate a supple spine and strong back. As age and decrepitude attempt to assert themselves, this pose is a superior tool to combat the insidious influences of neglect. Practice and rejoice in the reward of good health.

Cobra

If you've been plagued by a sore back, you may find that after practicing Cobra and the next pose, Locust, your back pain will fade away. This was my experience when I began to practice 20 years ago. Sore backs are often the product of improper forward bending. Without the counter action of an extending back bend, our backs get sore from repetitive forward bending.

Lifting the torso off the floor engages the back muscles that support the spine. Spinal resistance to gravity by activating these muscles cues the body to build bone density.

The abdominal organs, kidneys, and adrenal glands receive a wonderful massage as the breath plays through the architecture of the arched torso. The kidneys are the wastewater treatment plants of the body, responsible for cleansing the blood of toxins. This pose gives them a nice squeeze to assist them in their work. As we descend from the pose and release the squeeze, fresh blood floods in to wash toxins away.

If you're a coffee drinker, your adrenal glands will thank you for this pose, too. Caffeine, despite its benign reputation, is an addictive drug, and consumption can lead to adrenal exhaustion. Caffeine stimulates the adrenal glands to secrete adrenaline, that often-pleasant energy boost we get when we have a cup of coffee. However, too much caffeine can exhaust the adrenal glands and leave us feeling out-of-sorts. Cobra Pose delivers much-needed support to these often caffeine-beleaguered glands. Caffeine consumption should be kept low to moderate.

Locust

Now that we've begun to limber up and strengthen the back, let's continue with the action of recruiting the lower half of the body for Locust Pose.

Stage I

If your core is not as strong as you'd like it to be and this is the first movement therapy you've practiced for some time, **Half Locust Pose** is a good place to start. ■ Lie prone and rest with the forehead or chin on the mat. ■ Take a few full breaths as you ground your arms and legs into the floor. Feel the breath in your belly and

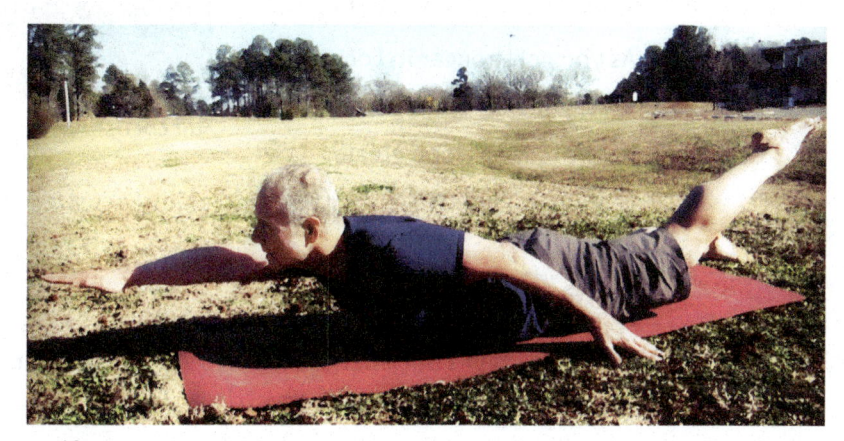

Half Locust Pose.

breathe smoothly. ■ **Simultaneously lift the head, chest, right arm, and left leg**. The right leg and left arm remain firmly grounded. The palm may be up or down for the grounded hand. **Lift strongly through the back and left leg.** ■ Breathe into the belly and fill the torso with breath. Hold the pose for several breaths or until fatigue gives you the cue to release your posture. Rest and relax. ■ Practice the posture on the other side.

Stage II

Lying prone, **simultaneously lift head, chest, and legs off the mat** just a few inches. You will immediately feel the full-body engagement of this posture. **Extend the arms to reach back along the side** and reach forward with the heart and torso and backwards with the buttocks and legs. Feel the length in this posture. **Breathe smoothly and deeply,** and notice how the breath

Locust

gives you a buoyant feeling in Locust Pose. Look ahead or down, whichever suits you. Hold the pose to the beginning of fatigue and slowly release and rest as you did in Cobra. As you get stronger in Locust Pose, you may extend the hands forward for a greater challenge. Please take your time and enjoy Locust.

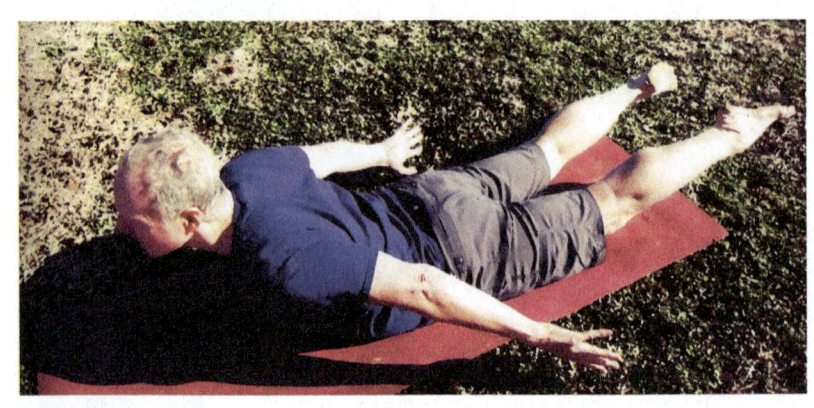

Full Locust Pose.

The Benefits

Even though this back bend is not as deep as Cobra, Locust Pose provides a different kind of engagement for the body. The organs and adrenals get much the same benefit, but the Locust goes a bit deeper into the core to massage and tone the abdominal organs and aorta, the artery that branches off to supply blood to the legs. This is sometimes the site for an aneurysm or a weak spot in this critical artery. Locust Pose will help tone and strengthen the aorta and all the abdominal organs.

Because this is a difficult pose, it builds perseverance and tenacity. The joy of persistent practice will be rewarded with noticeable endurance within a matter of days.

Nearly the entire body is resisting gravity in Locust Pose. This persistent resistance to gravity helps you to build your bones with each practice.

Locust Pose is also excellent for relieving sciatica and sacroiliac joint pain. Recently, I sustained a sacroiliac injury. Both the half and full Locust Poses were an important part of my recovery.

Plank

Plank Pose is probably most often practiced in yoga during a flow of poses called the Sun Salutation, but we'll practice it separately for our specific purposes.

Come down onto the ground onto all fours. Place the hands directly under the shoulders and the knees under the hips. ■ **Align the hands so the middle finger is aligned approximately between the two bones of the forearm. Flatten the palms and spread the fingers.** Flattening the palms and spreading the fingers gives the foundation of this pose lots of surface area for good support. Often students will simply dig the heels of the hands into the floor which causes the palms to rise without contacting the ground. This will lead to fatigue very quickly.

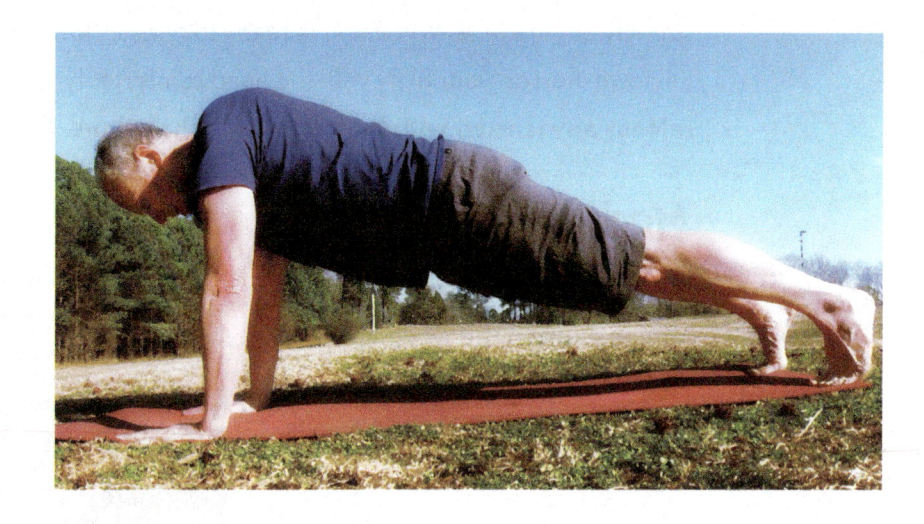

Push your feet back and lift the knees off the ground as if you were preparing for a pushup. ■ **Rotate the elbows so that the crook of the inner arm is facing forward.** ■ **Engage the shoulder muscles** by pushing the hands firmly into the ground. ■ Make sure that this pose is on **one flat plane**. Often students will raise the buttocks in order to make Plank Pose a bit easier. To get the full bone-density-building benefit from this pose, keep the body aligned in a flat plane.

Breathe deeply and maintain downward pressure with the hands. ■ Hold the pose and feel how gravity is working to pull you down. Resistance is what this pose is all about. Counteract this

Plank

gravitational pull with active hands, arms, shoulders, and feet. ■ Be conscious and mentally alert. Listen to your body. Feel what's happening throughout the bones and muscles that are so strongly engaged. ■ When you're ready to release, lower your knees to the ground and then lie down. Rest on your belly with the head comfortably positioned to either side. **Breathe and release any tension with long, mindful exhalations**. This is a simple but powerful pose.

Modification

If your wrists or elbows are not able to support the weight of your body in this pose, practice the following modification: from all fours, lower down onto your parallel forearms and elbows (or clasp your hands as pictured) and then push the feet back to straighten the knees. Adjust the elbows so that

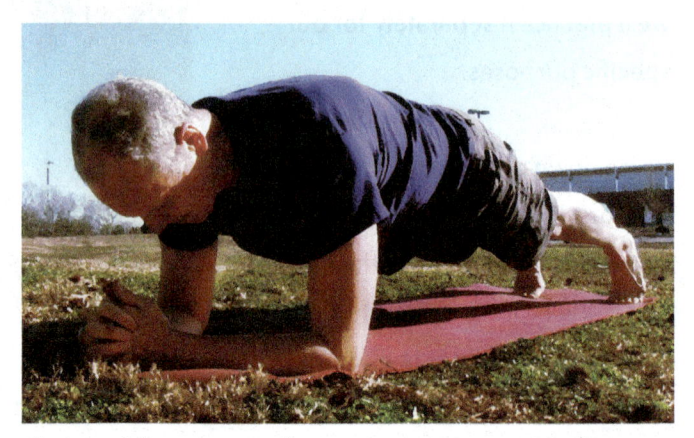

This modification puts less stress on wrists and elbows.

they are directly under the shoulders and the arms are parallel as you did for Cobra Stage II. You get all the benefits of this marvelous strength-building pose without the stress on the wrists and elbows.

The Benefits

Since the entire body is suspended on a flat plane, the spine, pelvis, and legs are all participating in a comprehensive posture that resists gravity. This posture strengthens hands, wrists, arms, shoulders, back, chest, and the core muscles of the abdomen, the pelvic girdle, and the legs. As this Plank Pose challenges you to build your strength, you will also develop greater willpower and perseverance. Plank Pose is a full-body bone-building posture.

Bridge

The inventors of the ancient science of Hatha Yoga were astute scholars of physics and body mechanics. They realized and practiced the dynamic oppositional forces that can be readily channeled by using the body, breath, and gravity. Bridge Pose is a good example of this knowledge.

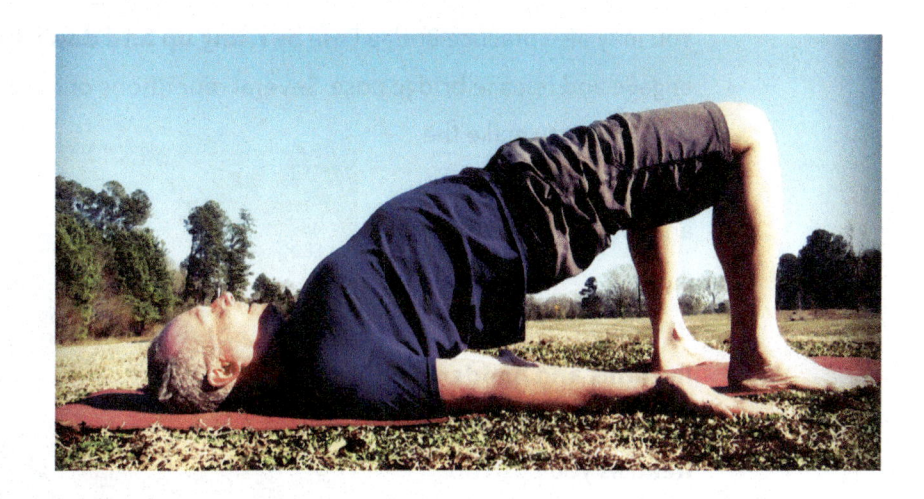

Begin by lying on your back. ■ Take some nice, full, restful breaths. ■ With the arms lying along the sides, palms up or down, **push into your feet**. Feel how this grounds the shoulder blades. ■ **Lift the buttocks and back off the ground** slowly and evenly. ■ As you reach the peak of your ascent, **gently push the chin into the top of the breast bone** where it connects to the collar bones. ■ Now, **gently push your head into the floor** to engage your neck muscles and the cervical spine at the base of the skull. This activates the entire neck and throat to help build bone density.

Feel the wonderful arch in the back created by this bridge architecture. ■ **Draw the breath deeply into this shape**. ■ **Use the diaphragm to push the breath strongly into the navel and sacrum at the base of the spine**. This is one of the greatest self massages in all of Hatha Yoga. ■ Hold Bridge Pose and use the full breath to realize the maximum benefit. ■ When you get the inner cue, **release the pose slowly** as you land each vertebrae separately until you touch the sacrum to the ground. ■ Snuggle your back into the mat and savor the results of this invigorating back bend.

Modifications

You may also practice Bridge Pose by **rising up and down in a slow wave-like motion** as you engage and release bridge pose. Several repetitions of this flowing motion will loosen up the back and may make the sustained pose easier and more comfortable.

In another variation, the **arms and hands sweep up above the head** as you push up into the pose. When you reach the peak of the pose, ground the arms into the floor and feel the little extra upward boost you get from pressing the arms downward.

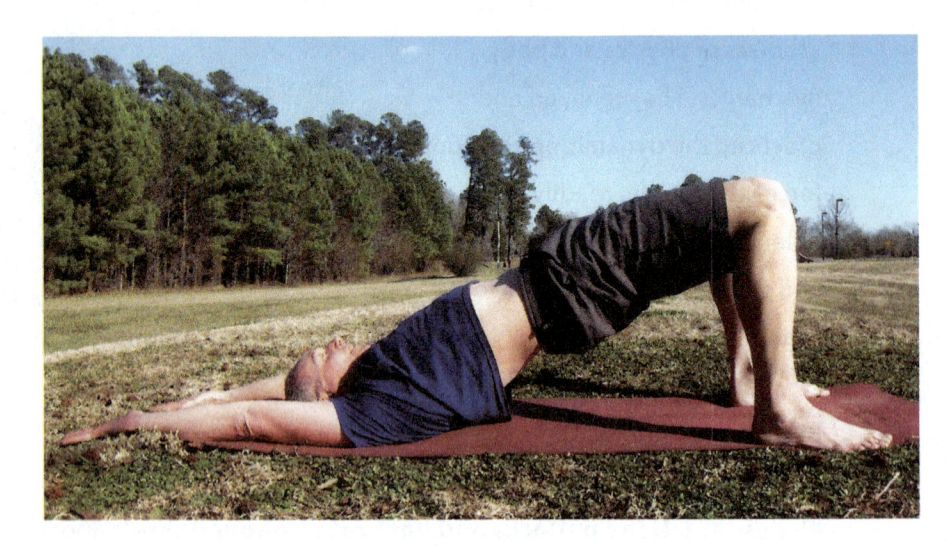

As you develop strength and mastery in Bridge Pose and would like to challenge yourself a bit more, try this strong modification: when you are at the zenith of the pose, **clasp the hands together under the body**. Walk the shoulders under the body one at a time by leaning over on one side and pulling the opposite shoulder under and then pulling the other shoulder under. This adds a robust chest-opening dimension to this already powerful pose.

The Benefits

The feet and upper back exert leverage that forces the back off the ground into the shape of a bridge. The gluteus and back muscles are strongly activated to support this architecture. The posterior spine, as with all the back bends, receives a deep compression as the front of the spine opens up to decompress the vertebrae. The architecture of Bridge Pose is one of the very best ways for the spine to resist gravity and build bone density.

For those of us past our mid-twenties, spinal flexion and extension is vital in keeping the spine supple. Even in the youth of our late twenties, according to anatomist David Coulter, author of *Anatomy of Hatha Yoga*, the capillaries in the disks begin to dry up. It is theorized that the disks must then absorb blood from the vertebrae directly. The back-bending poses are essential to healthy aging of the spine because they facilitate flexibility through enhanced circulation and disposal of waste products.

As the chin presses down onto the sternum, the thyroid and parathyroid glands are also compressed and massaged by the deep breath. This stimulates these glands to balance their hormone production and help regulate a healthy immune system.

The posterior portions of the lungs and heart also receive a deep massaging compression. The front of the heart gets a good massage as it pushes up against the sternum.

For the brain, this pose is a bit of an inversion, so blood is flowing into the skull because of gravity. As you see, there is a lot going on in Bridge Pose—and it's all good!

Boat

Boat pose is an often-avoided posture in yoga practice because it demands so much from the core. Yes, it's a hard pose. This is how the body shows us the good work that we really need to do to. Anytime we encounter a particularly difficult pose, we discover muscles that need strengthening.

To encourage you to practice this powerful pose, let me give you a great example of a woman with a "boat" load of strength. Ida Herbert is a 96-year-old yoga teacher who can hold boat pose for five solid minutes. Though I lay claim to being a fairly accomplished Hatha Yogi myself, I can't come close to this great feat of endurance. Let us all take courage from Ida's example and get started building our core strength and bone density.

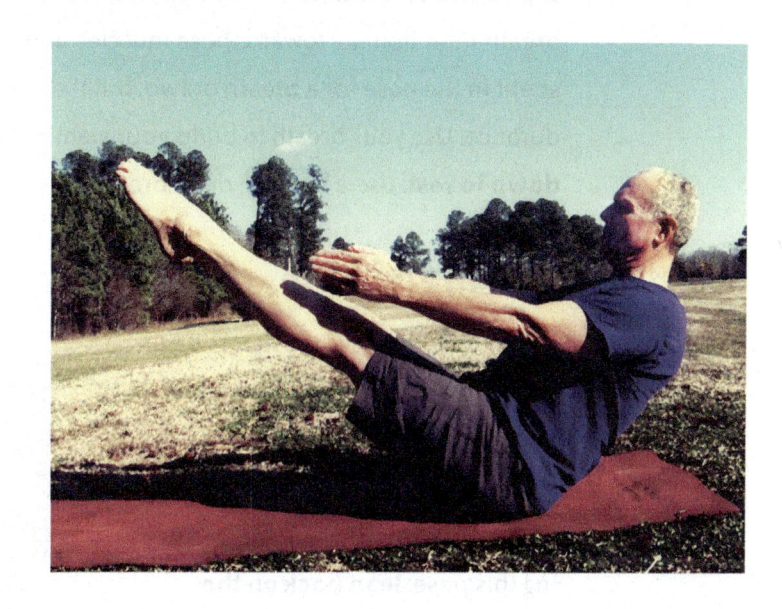

Begin by sitting with the legs flat on the floor in front of you, arms beside you, pushing your palms into the floor with the fingertips pointing forward. ■ **Snuggle the sitting bones into the ground** as you compose your concentration with full, conscious breaths. ■ From this stable platform, **lean back to about 45 degrees**. ■ Using the hands to support you, **lift the legs up a few inches**. Remember, no straining. Just an inch will be enough to engage your core muscles and the portions of the spine to which they attach. ■ The hands may remain at the sides or, **if you are ready for a bit more of a challenge, raise the arms** like an airplane or reach them forward.

Boat

Use the full three-part breath to help ground and stabilize your posture. Keep drawing in full, supportive breaths. ■ As you begin to tire, notice where the fatigue is and try to focus your breath intentionally toward those muscles and see if that helps. It may only increase your time spent in the pose for a breath or two, but it shows you the power of the breath to increase endurance. Use your breath to build your stamina and determination. ■ **Slowly release and lie down to rest.** Use a few full, deep breaths to dissipate any lingering tension.

Modifications

If raising both legs is too much, begin with one leg at a time and slowly build your endurance. If your back still feels strained, here is a great way to support the back while learning this pose: **lean back on the arms with the elbows bent** and the forearms and hands as your support structure—just like you were hanging out at the beach. Then raise one or both legs off the ground to engage Boat Pose. **Point your toes**, tuck the heels, contract the Achilles tendons that connect the heel to lower calf muscle, and pull the knee caps up firmly. Remember, you're in no hurry. Even the gentlest form of any pose will begin the process of strengthening your muscles and bones.

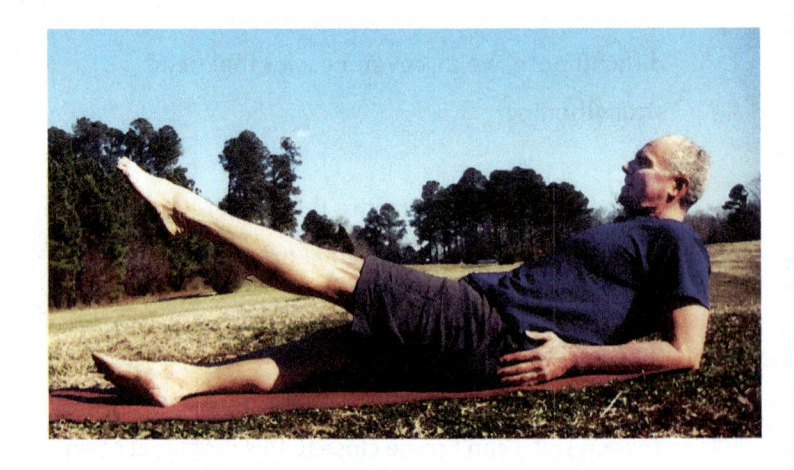

The Benefits

Boat Pose engages the low back and the abdominal core muscles. The entire spine is engaged from top to bottom in bone-building resistance to gravity. Even a short stay in Boat Pose helps you feel this very quickly. The muscles throughout the front of the pelvis and on the top and inside of the thighs also get a nice toning workout in Boat Pose.

Yoga Sit-Ups

Before you groan in protest, allow me to say that these techniques can be executed with ease or vigor. It's up to you. Even the easiest way works. So, **take it easy at first** and build your strength slowly and enjoyably! Soon, with a bit of effort, you'll be proud of how much stronger you have become.

Lie flat on your back and relax with a few nice cleansing breaths. See, how hard was that? ■ **Draw the feet up behind the buttocks**, hip-width apart with the knees bent, feet on the ground, or raise the legs straight up at a 90-degree angle to the body. ■ **Put your hands behind your head**, intertwine the fingers, and cradle the head into the palms of the hands to support your neck. ■ Inhale. ■ As you begin your exhalation, slowly raise the shoulder blades off the ground just a few inches. ■ **Curl the lower spine inward** as you engage the abdominal muscles to **pull the sacrum up as well**. If your sacrum doesn't make it all the way off the ground, don't worry about it. As you gain strength, your sacrum will begin to rise in small increments. Hold until you exhale and lie back down while inhaling. Not so bad, huh? ■ **Go at your own pace** and practice three sets of five to begin with, or whatever you feel you're capable of SAFELY accomplishing.

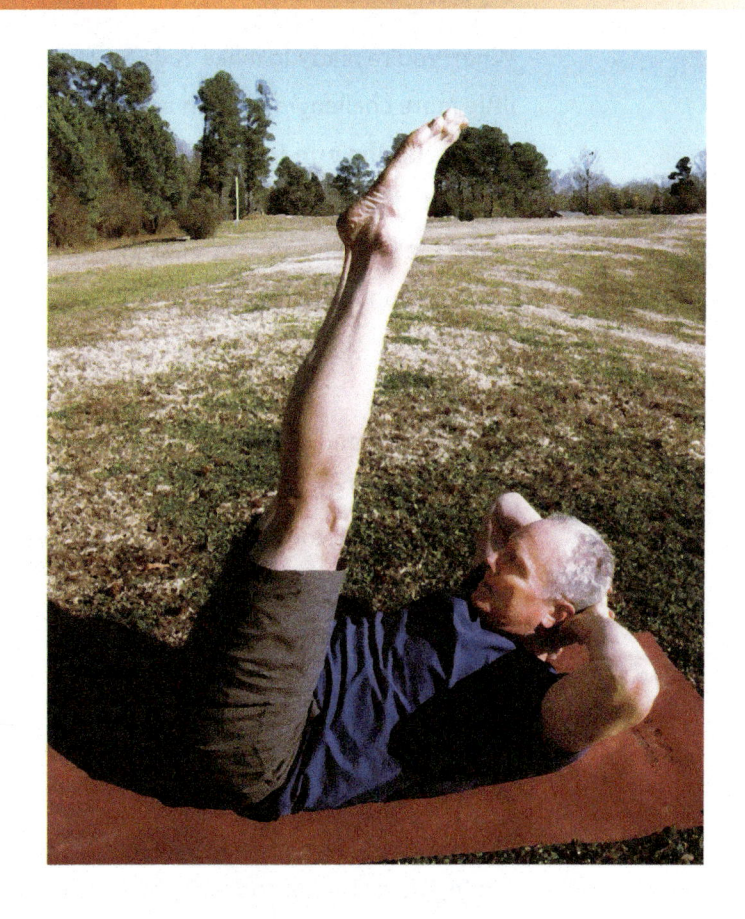

Yoga Sit-Ups

Modification

When you're ready to make Yoga Sit-Ups a little more challenging, **reach across your body with the arm to the outside of the opposite knee**. With this crossover technique the sacrum and lower back remain on the ground. Again, take it easy. Enjoy yourself.

Begin slowly, and gently work toward a higher level of strength and fortitude. As you become more accomplished in this empowering practice, your confidence and self-esteem will grow.

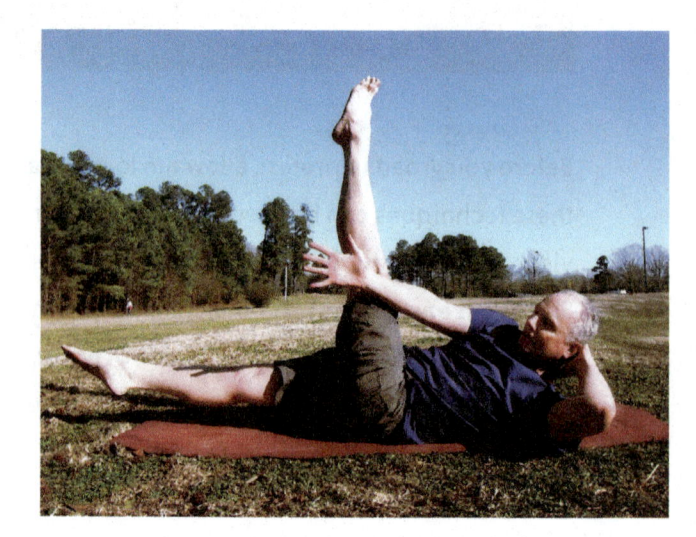

The Benefits

Unlike Boat Pose, you get to rest between each repetition. This way the muscles, bones, and connective tissue can safely participate in these sit-ups.

Again, the resistance to gravity helps your bone tissue get denser each time you practice.

The abdominal muscles, back, and neck are all strengthened by sit-ups. I especially like reaching across the body until I begin to feel the burn of exertion. This is a good signal to rest.

Each sit-up repetition massages the abdominal organs and stretches and tones the kidneys and adrenal glands.

With the legs aloft, this posture aids in returning blood to the heart as gravity pulls it back down.

Savasana

Savasana is the traditional resting pose after a yoga session. Savasana means **Corpse Pose**, which may seem like a rather macabre term. The idea is to lie completely still in conscious relaxation. You may even feel more relaxed than you would after sleeping. Conscious, intentional rest produces deep healing and rejuvenation.

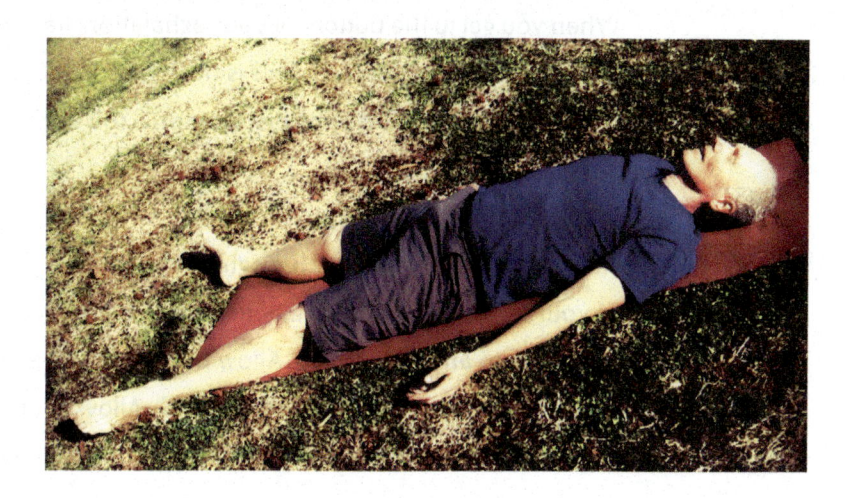

How is that possible you might ask? And why is this necessary? Conscious relaxation can produce a more deeply relaxed state than sleep. In sleep, we may grind our teeth, dream, and then respond with subsequent tension. In conscious relaxation, we deliberately rest each region of the body and surrender utterly to gravity. Fifteen minutes spent in Savasana can provide relaxation worth hours of sleep.

Relaxation after exertion allows the body to collate and incorporate the physical and mental hygiene that is accomplished in our Hatha Yoga practice. Hygiene may seem an odd word choice, but I use it to denote the conscious, fastidious attention to the body that is uncommon but so necessary to promote good health and strong bones. This is the kind of attention and awareness that we cultivate in a regular yoga practice.

Conscious, intentional rest produces deep healing and rejuvenation.

So take your rest and gain the enormous benefit.

Savasana

Lie down on your back with your hands and legs about 45 degrees out from the center line of your body. ■ Slowly drink in several deep, full three-part breaths and release them slowly. ■ When you get to the bottom of your exhalation, lie completely still and **suspend the breath for a few moments if you can**. This is the essence of Corpse Pose—no breath, no motion. ■ **Bathe in the stillness of that sublime moment**. You may use breath suspension after every breath if you like.

As you resume your breath, begin at the soles of your feet and consciously relax each part of your body. ■ If you feel any residual tension from your day or from your practice, **breathe deeply into any tense area**. Allow the inhalation to massage the tense area and then feel the tension dissipate with the exhalation. ■ Allow your body to drape itself over the ground and fully surrender to gravity. ■ Remain conscious and watch your body slowly relax.

Even though you are alert and awake, allow the mind to rest as well. Savasana becomes a lying-down meditation. **In order to keep the mind alert** and connected to your breath, you may want to use a simple mantra. If so, "blue sky—white clouds" is emotionally evocative. As you inhale say to yourself, "blue sky," and as you exhale internally chant, "white clouds." Feel your body becoming more and more relaxed with each breath cycle.

Rest for as long as you like; the longer the better. ■ **When you're ready to resume your day**, slowly begin to deepen your breath, gently wiggle fingers and toes, and take a gentle inhaling stretch with the hands over the head ■ **As you exhale, slowly roll over to either side**, use your shoulder for a pillow if you don't have one handy, and continue to rest.

I call this **Providence Pose** because I always feel, for some reason, that everything I need will be provided for me. If this resonates for you, luxuriate in the affirmation that you are building denser, stronger bones. Smile.

Savasana

Slowly, slowly, rise to a comfortable sitting position. ■ Allow your head to droop forward as you rise. ■ As you slowly lift your chin, feel the blood drain from your skull and sit quietly for a few minutes enjoying the equanimity you've gained through your practice and rest. ■ Now, consciously breathe your way into motion with gratitude and joy.

I can never say this enough: be gentle and take it easy. Resist the social conditioning to make this joyful practice strenuous or competitive. Practicing gently and consistently will give you the best results. You'll be surprised.

One of our great founding fathers, Thomas Jefferson, counseled friends to always "take life by the smooth handle." He could just as easily have been talking about yoga. Life is stressful enough. Strenuous workouts can contribute to high cortisol levels in the blood. Cortisol is a stress-response hormone that revs the body up for fight or flight. Chronically high levels of cortisol contribute to hypertension. High levels of cortisol also suppress the immune system and decrease bone formation.

> *Resist the social conditioning to make this joyful practice strenuous or competitive. Practicing gently and consistently will give you the best results.*

Practicing in a diligent but relaxed fashion helps diffuse tension and lower blood pressure. I call Hatha Yoga practice an exorcism of the tension demons. *The Dynamic Dozen* and all the other wonderful postures of Hatha Yoga, along with the deep three-part breath, help release tension and return our biochemistry to its normal state. Regular practice keeps the body free of excess tension and stress that accumulates in our tissues. This is just one of the marvelous ways in which Hatha Yoga prevents disease.

A relaxed being is a being that is capable of healing and restoring the body to vibrant health—a being that is able to rebuild bone density.

Savasana

I wish you joy and abundant health as you practice *The Dynamic Dozen*. You are at the beginning of what may be the greatest adventure of your life: The journey to the center of yourself.

> You are at the beginning of what may be the greatest adventure of your life: The journey to the center of yourself

Yoga teaches us that we are divine beings whose true nature is bliss. Our worldly experience teaches us quite the opposite. Use this infinitely powerful practice to begin your journey back to who you really are. You are strong, powerful, relaxed, and blissful.

Namaste,

Tim

Acknowledgements

It is with love and gratitude that I thank my beautiful partner, **Michele Tracy Berger**, for her constant encouragement to write. I've always had an ambivalent relationship to writing, never thinking that anything I could write would ever make much of a difference. "Who cares what I've got to say," was my ready refrain to any inclination about writing. Ah, the deceptive, discouraging voice of the inner critic. But I have learned that if we communicate from our hearts, there will be an audience who wants to hear what we have to say.

Thanks to **Marjorie Hudson** and **Melissa Delbridge**, my writing teachers. They both created a nurturing atmosphere and always offered gentle, constructive guidance that supported my fledgling flights into the wild blue yonder of writing.

Thanks also to **Liz Moudy (Saranpreet Kaur)**. She was my first reader and helped me begin the process of shaping this book.

Resources

- *Anatomy of Hatha Yoga: A Manual for Students, Teachers, and Practitioners* by H. David Coulter (Body and Breath)

- *The Heart of Yoga: Developing a Personal Practice* by T.K.V. Desikachar (Inner Traditions/Bear & Company)

- *Yoga Mind, Body and Spirit : A Return to Wholeness* by Donna Farhi (Holt, Henry & Company, Inc.)

- *Yoga: The Spirit and Practice of Moving into Stillness* by Erich Schiffman (Gallery Books)

- *A.M. Yoga for Your Week* with Rodney Yee (video available at Gaiam.com)

CPSIA information can be obtained
at www.ICGtesting.com
Printed in the USA
LVOW02s1013230217
525201LV00005B/85/P

9 780991 150250